Science, Spirituality and Evolution

Published by
Mzuni Press
P/Bag 201 Luwinga
Mzuzu 2

ISBN 978-99960-60-30-4
eISBN 978-99960-60-31-1

Mzuni Texts no. 7

The Mzuni Press is represented outside Africa by:
African Books Collective Oxford (order@africanbookscollective.com)

www.mzunipress.blogspot.com

www.africanbookscollective.com

Science, Spirituality
and
Evolution

John A. Ryan

Mzuni Texts no. 7

Mzuni Press

Mzuzu

2017

Table of Contents

Introduction

I feel excited. As a priest in the Catholic Church, I have had a wonderful opportunity of promoting the Spiritual in our lives for over 30 years now. As a person who enjoys Mathematics I have had the joy of passing on this passion to others. Sometimes people ask me 'how did you as a Missionary Priest get so heavily involved in promoting Mathematics?' I answer something like 'The Mission to spread the Kingdom of God and the Mission of passing on a passion for Mathematics is the same for me'. I emphasise *for me*. For others, it could be hospital work, for yet others it could be building churches, etc etc. God has deposited a variety of gifts in his people and he expects each to use their gifts for the building up of His Kingdom.

The beauty and elegance found in Mathematics has always pointed me to the Divine and, in my own mind, I never saw any division. However, it was not always easy to communicate this 'oneness' to others. Now, for the first time, with the elegant mathematics involved in the Quantum World, it is becoming easier to communicate some of the riches and wonderment exposed to one who pursues Mathematics. In the same process, the apparent divide which has existed between Science and Religion is being obliterated. The exciting element is that, it is possible to communicate a lot of this in non-technical terms and so make it accessible to the non-mathematician and to a far wider audience. I do hope that the reader will be enriched by the following pages.

Chapter 1: Science versus Religion

1.   The Clash of Science and Religion

The Institute of Electrical and Electronic Engineers[1] (IEEE) is one of
the largest and most respected professional bodies in the scientific
world and Spectrum Radio[2] is its official on-line radio station. On
Spectrum Radio, in April 2009, Steven Cherry interviewed Robert
Park who is Professor of Physics at the University of Maryland in
the USA about his views on Science and Belief in God. In the
interview Park says

> What troubles me the most is the fact that some
> scientists are believers. I find that very hard to
> understand. That you can be a scientist and
> compartmentalize your beliefs so thoroughly—on the
> one side you use one set of rules to draw conclusions
> and then on the other side you use an entirely
> different set of rules, a contradictory set of rules, to
> draw other conclusions.

Robert Park is a product of the education system during the latter
half of the twentieth century where Science and Religion mis-
understood each other. Science and Religion seemed to be
disciplines belonging to different worlds. Many people, like Robert
Park, felt that they were irreconcilable. In this paper, we show how
Science and Religion are now coming to the same conclusions
using different paths.

_____

[1]   http://www.ieee.org/
[2]   http://spectrum.ieee.org/

2.   The Logic behind the Clash

It is clear that Robert Park expects everything to follow the same set of rules, the same set of logical argument and the same route as mapped out by the physical laws of science, by the Law of Gravity, by Newton's Laws of Motion, by Boyle's Law for Gases etc. One set of rules applies to all of reality. One set of rules explains all of reality. One set of rules directs all of reality. One set of rules fits all.

The set of rules that Robert Park is talking about originates from the systematic deductive logic as first developed by Aristotle who was born in 384 BC and died in 322 BC.[3] Aristotle believed that logic is the basis of all Science and he was the first to propose that each branch of Science should begin with its own set of axioms, an accepted set of principles from which everything else is deduced. Aristotle himself did not use the term 'logic' but talked about 'analytics' and developed the famous 'Prior Analytics' which consists of two premises and a conclusion as in the following example, which was given by Aristotle himself:

- Every Greek is a person
- Every person is mortal
  Therefore every Greek is mortal.[4]

This systematic deductive logic became supreme in all of scientific thought, scientific investigation and scientific development. Science here is used in its widest sense, including disciplines like Sociology and Philosophy. Aristotle also saw logic as uniting all of knowledge and saw mathematics, philosophy and physics as

---

[3]   http://www.bookrags.com/biography/aristotle/
[4]   http://ebooks.adelaide.edu.au/a/aristotle/a8pra/

different faces of one reality. Aristotle did not separate different scientific disciplines into different boxes but realised that all areas of life were connected and interconnected. Plato's Academy,[5] which Aristotle helped to develop, was not only devoted to mathematics and science but also philosophy, religion and politics, as all were seen as related. However, it is in more recent times that knowledge was boxed and parcelled in separate compartments and as Science tried to specialize more and more, this compartmentalization reached its extreme.

On the other hand, Robert Park sees 'Belief in God' as belief on the basis of submission to a higher authority with no reference to logical argument or rational discourse. For him such a 'Belief' is 'ill-informed'. An entirely 'different set of rules' is applied in its justification. The fact that such a 'Belief in God' cannot be 'objectively proven beyond doubt' using systematic deductive logic is a problem for him. The 'Belief in God' does not stand up to the scrutiny of scientific investigation which follows one set of rules which include the laws of deductive logic, Newton's Laws of Motion, Boyle's Law for Gases etc. For Robert Park, everything has to follow this one set of rules.

We are merely taking Robert Park as an example of the all too common position taken by many in the academic world during the latter part of the last century when 'Belief in God' was often seen as incompatible with scientific experiment and scientific rigour.[6] But this need not be the case.

---

[5]   http://en.wikipedia.org/wiki/Platonic_Academy.
[6]   John Polkinghorne, *Quantum Physics and Theology*, Yale University Press, 2007.

Chapter 2: Science

1.   The Building Blocks of All Matter

The process of compartmentalisation of knowledge was given
great impetus by another concept which crept into scientific
thought and research, namely the idea of breaking down a thing
into its constituent parts and seeing an entity as merely the sum of
its parts. Full knowledge of a thing could be gained by breaking it
down into simpler parts, knowing the makeup of the simpler parts
and then putting the parts together to make the whole. This
model works well for a machine or a computer. Computer repair,
in fact, is merely about identifying one of the six or seven parts of a
computer which is not functioning properly and then replacing that
part. The model works well for a bicycle. Again, identify the part
giving problems, replace it and the bicycle is ready again for
cycling. It is this very model which motivated scientists to search
for the basic building blocks of all matter. Perhaps this idea came
originally from Plato who believed everything was made from four
elements, namely earth, fire, air and water. [7] They were referred
to as the 'Platonic solids'. By the beginning of the twentieth
century, this list was replaced by another list of 103 elements
which were considered indivisible and all matter was constituted
from these 103 elements.[8] Again, the idea was that full
understanding of matter could be gained by breaking it down into
its constituent parts. Emphasis is placed on full knowledge of the
individual parts. Then simply adding up or putting together the
well known and well researched individual parts gives rise to full
knowledge of matter in its different forms. Therefore, much effort

---

[7]   http://en.wikipedia.org/wiki/Platonic_solids.

[8]   http://www.periodic-table.com/.

is placed on isolating the individual parts and attaining 'full knowledge' about them and of them.

2. Scientific Method

This 'isolating individual parts' or 'extracting specific situations' has been the approach of Science in all its forms up to the present day. First, one isolates a situation, puts restrictions and clearly defined limits on it and then analyses it in minute detail and in depth. This method has been applied not only in the Empirical Sciences but also in the Social Sciences, in Philosophy, in Theology and in many life situations. It is an effort to simplify life situations and bring them to manageable portions which can then be analysed and controlled. It is an effort to be in charge of life situations, to be able to manipulate and dominate the processes of life. This was epitomised by the French mathematician, Pierre Laplace, in the 19th century when he said:

> An intelligence knowing all forces acting in nature as well as knowing the positions of all things—to it nothing would be uncertain, both future and past would be present before its eyes. [9]

In the last couple of centuries this linear logic and this scientific method of breaking things down into smaller and simpler parts was seen as the tool not only for understanding all of reality but for fixing all problems and for making progress in all of life situations.

3. Objectivity in Science

Objective truth has become the bedrock of all progress where having isolated a situation, definite 'objective' conclusions are

---

[9]   Quoted in *Superforce* by Paul Davies, London Unwin Books, 1984.

derived and these 'objective' conclusions are given a prominence and a permanency that is associated with the word 'objective'. Intuition and imagination have no role to play in serious science or in serious research. Everything has to be 'objective' and 'proven beyond doubt' in order to gain the respect of the scientific community. Everything has to follow the linear logic of Aristotle and fit in with the Law of Gravity or Newton's Laws of Motion or Boyle's Law etc. "Rational" is the word which must apply to all scientific investigation if it is to be credible or accepted by the scientific community or if it is to be accepted as 'objective'.

4. The Benefits Science Brought

There is no doubt that such 'objective' science has brought benefits to humankind on planet Earth. Especially in Western Europe and in the United States of America as well as in other 'developed' countries, the drudgery has been taken out of the daily struggle to feed, clothe and house oneself with the result of much longer life spans for many. Mechanisation in farming has increased food production several times over. Motor cars and airplanes, roads and airports have made travel easy and comfortable. The advances in telecommunications in recent years have allowed us to be in constant contact with one another despite being physically separated by big distances. Television, radio and iPods are opening up many opportunities and possibilities for humans. The list goes on and on. We could easily fill pages describing the benefits brought to humankind by Science. Notice I say 'benefits to **humankind'**, I am not claiming any benefits for animals or for the flowers, for the forests, for the rivers, for the wetlands, for the seas, for the fish, for the birds, for the air etc.

5. The Misery that Science Brought

But Science has also brought misery and destruction to some of humankind. The thirst to dominate and control, as inspired by Science, has given way to much war and strife. The proliferation of arms in the world, especially in the less developed countries, is giving rise to a lot of crime and insecurity. Weapons of mass destruction have not only decimated large populations with continuing cancerous and deadly infections for present and future generations but are also a constant threat to our survival on planet Earth. Drugs, modern technology and greed have brought great sophistication into crime throughout the developed world posing great challenges to policing and law enforcing agents. Children can no longer roam freely in playful abandonment but have to be constantly supervised by known and trusted adults. Population explosion is also posing huge challenges. At the present rate of population growth, a billion people are being added to planet Earth every 30 years. For the first time ever, the continent of Africa is now supporting one billion people. This together with climate change, deforestation, depletion of soils, droughts, use of chemicals etc, is perpetuating and propagating further poverty and misery in many people's lives. The exploitation of women, human trafficking and prostitution are increasing at alarming rates everywhere throughout the world through the various means of modern technology. Young minds are being poisoned with pornography both in print and electronic forms. The air, the rivers, the seas, the mountains, the plains, the lakes, the wetlands, the bogs etc, are being polluted with toxic chemicals due to modern methods of farming and mass industrial means of production. The list goes on and on.

It is the same mechanistic model of Science and the same Aristotelian logic which is allowing the rich to become richer at the expense of the poor. The economic gap between those who are accumulating vast material resources for themselves and those who live on the edge in isolated areas of the world is widening. Those who are doing the accumulating for themselves are changing the climate in isolated areas resulting (for example in some cases) in drought where essential crops fail, giving rise to poverty, sicknesses, starvation and death. And then when the international aid agencies come in with emergency help, which is not only necessary but essential, the spirit of self reliance is destroyed and replaced by a dependency syndrome further perpetuating the economic inequity. Those who leave the isolation of rural areas and congregate in urban ghettos, suffer not only from economic inequities but also from social inequities. The scale and experience of inequity is exacerbated giving rise to even more social problems. The list goes on and on.

Chapter 3: Spirituality, Religion and Theology

Let us begin this chapter by exploring what we mean by the three terms (a) Spirituality, (b) Religion and (c) Theology.

a. Spirituality is the quest for meaning in life. It is inherent in the human condition. It asks the major life questions like: Where did we come from? Where are we going? What is the meaning of life? What am I here for? Humans have grappled with these questions from the beginning of human history, nearly 100,000 years ago.   When our ancient ancestors offered sacrifices to the gods in the mountains or in the forests they were taking part in this quest for meaning in life. We are still grappling with these questions today. The search takes many and varied forms. Many search within the established religions and churches. Others search outside these structures. When people climb Kaning'ina mountain to pray all night they are partaking in this very search. When people gather together to sing, dance and speak in tongues they are also partaking in this search. Some would say the indulging in drugs, sex and alcohol is a misguided effort in this search, an effort which of course only leads to destruction and emptiness. Spirituality is as varied as there are people and as old as humanity itself.

b. Religion, on the other hand, is a recent visitor to our planet. All the major religions have their origins within the last 5,000 years. Different religions may have very different origins but, in general, Religion does organise, direct and shape Spirituality, it gives it a context within which to express it, to celebrate it and explore it further. Some have observed that the major religions came within the period of the agricultural revolution (the last 10,000 years) when planet earth was divided up and further divided and subdivided into different countries, regions, districts, estates, farms etc and when boundaries and borders were constructed and peoples claimed ownership and sovereignity over parcels of land and water. The advent of religions came within the era of this parcelling and subdividing and ordering of property and agriculture and livelihoods. O'Murchu poses the question: "Was Religion also an effort to organise and even control spirituality?"[10]

c. The word 'Theology' comes from the two Latin words 'Theos' meaning God and 'Logos' meaning word. In Christian circles, at least up to 1200 AD, theology was mainly about interpreting the Bible and in particular the four Gospels of the New Testament within the tradition of the Christian Church founded by Jesus. Theology was seen as bringing out the deeper meaning of these books and their practical implications for daily life of the Christian faithful. Around the thirteenth century Thomas Acquinas broadened this understanding of Theology saying Theology

---

[10] Diarmud O'Murchu, *Quantum Theology* , Crossroad Publishing, New York, 2004, Chapter 2.

was 'Faith Seeking Understanding'. Then, after the Reformation period and the establishment of the Protestant Churches, the Protestant Churches continued an allegiance to the Bible as the supreme authority while the Catholic Church developed a sacramental and canonical approach. Theology then was developed as particular traditions within particular churches giving rise to different theologies.

1. Recent Developments in Theology[11]

In more recent times the focus of Theology was further broadened with the recovery of the real meaning of the term 'Word' as translated from the Hebrew 'Dabhar'; Dabhar meaning that Divine Creative Energy which was there from the beginning. In the beginning of John's Gospel, we read "In the beginning was the Word and the Word was with God and the Word was God." The 'Word' here has a very rich meaning — that Divine Creative Intelligence, Creative Wisdom, Creative Energy, which was there in the beginning, there throughout all of the billions of years of history of the universe, continually creating, continually shaping, continually transforming and still there now continuing to create, shape and transform everything. St Paul says "All of creation is groaning in one great act of giving birth."[12] The churches continually talk about 'saving and renewing' bringing about a 'new heaven and a new earth'. So Theology now is seen as exploring that Divine Dabhar which continues to create, to sustain and to transform. Theology is no longer the preserve of any one church

---

[11] Diarmud O'Murchu, *Quantum Theology* , Crossroad Publishing, New York, 2004, Chapter 2.
[12] Romans 8:22

or one tradition but now even explores ways and means of bringing all these diverse traditions closer together, recognizing that no one tradition contains all the wisdom but that the fuller picture is found in the diversity of all traditions. So in recent times different strains of Theology have emerged. Among the different strains are:

a. Liberation Theology: A Christian Theology more about liberation in this world than salvation in a life to come. It is very pragmatic, it considers the system and the structural oppression and it seeks political change and changes in the structure. It is not a top down approach but begins with human beings in their daily life struggle.

b. Feminist Theology: It is not just about ordination of women but treats far more fundamental questions and challenges patriarchy and sexism. It seeks to overcome the traditional dualism of emotions vs intellect, heart vs head, irrational vs rational. The emphasis is on being holistic, inclusive and in harmony.

c. Creation Theology: Traditionally theology considered the world to be a transitory place, not worthy of deep trust and love. The world was identified with planet Earth. The 'End of the World' loomed large in traditional theology. Now we are far more knowledgable about the origins of not only planet Earth but of the whole universe, we are invited to confront our anthropocentrism (seeing things only from the human point of view), we realize that we share this world and this universe with many other creatures, we are invited to examine our 'world denouncing spirituality', to reverse our 'masculine tendencies to dominate', to halt the 'manipulation and the exploitation of creation' for human benefit. We are invited to see the bigger picture, our place in that bigger picture and thus bow down in respect and homage before it all.

d. Inter-Church Theology: Inter-Church Theology is raising many intruiging questions. All religions are attempts to interpret and contextualize God's revelation to Humanity. The possibility that religions belong to the Age of Patriarchy and to the Age of the Agricultural Revolution (8,000 BC -2,000 AD) and may have diminished importance as we move into a new evolutionary epoc may need to be examined further in the light of the present decline of religious practice in many parts of the 'developed' world. In the past Religion was the main way in which people explored and articulated their spiritual desires while today people are doing it in other ways.

Chapter 4: What is Quantum?

1.   Our Limited Vision

We live in a world which we experience with our five senses of hearing, seeing, smelling, tasting and touching. We are limited by these five senses. A fish that lives its whole life in water has no idea and no picture of what the lake looks like from the mountains. The fish probably cannot even imagine what is not water. The fact that it lives all its life in water limits its understanding to 'water things' and it has no idea of what is 'outside water'. We humans are no different. We literally find it difficult to see 'beyond our noses'. We are limited because we can only 'see' with our ears, eyes, nose, tongue (to taste) and hand (to touch). We cannot see that space and time are just different sides of one thing and maybe not even different sides but as Einstein said just 'one continuum'—the space time continuum, something which is far bigger than what we can imagine, something which envelops us and envelops our whole world. And since we live all our lives 'in the water' we are unable to see the mountains and unable to see the lake from the mountains. We are unable to see and experience the space time continuum.

Nor can we see or feel or smell or taste or touch the smallest pieces of matter which make up our bodies and make up the world we live in. We only experience the 'middle world', the world which consists of:

- things which are far bigger than atoms and electrons (those things which we can experience, can see, can touch, can smell, can taste, can hear) and

- things which are far smaller than the larger realities like the space time continuum.

2.   Three Levels of World

We have then three realities or three levels of world:

1.   The Microscopic World made up of quarks, electrons, atoms etc. The Microscopic World is real but not immediately accessible to our senses.
2.   The Middle World made up of things which we can experience and where we exist. The Middle World is available to our senses.
3.   The Macro World which envelops us. The Macro World is real but not immediately accessible to our senses.

3.   The Quantum World

Quantum is about the Microscopic World. Quantum Physics explores the realities of the microscopic world. Quantum Mechanics tries to manipulate the microscopic world. Quantum Mathematics describes the microscopic world. Quantum Theology explores the spiritual implications of the new knowledge of the microscopic world. Entering into the microscopic world is entering a world unknown to us, a world which (despite the fact that it provides the building blocks of all of reality as we know it) does not obey the laws of the middle world. It is a world which baffles us. It is a world which does not follow 'our logic'. It is a world of mystery. It is a world of fascination. It is beyond our understanding, beyond our dreams and beyond our imaginings. Niels Bohr, who won the Nobel Prize for Physics in 1922, said "He who is not shocked by the Quantum World does not understand it."[13] We are only beginning to realise how mysterious it all is. Yet entering into the microscopic world gives us a better under-standing of the middle world. It in fact changes our 'world view'.

---

[13] http://nobelprize.org/nobel_prizes/physics/laureates/1922/bohr-bio.html

Chapter 5: Mathematics and the Quantum

1.   Some Thoughts on Mathematics

Some confuse mathematics with numbers. Numbers are used in many disciplines, e.g. accountancy, engineering, history, geography, and mathematics is just another discipline where numbers are sometimes used. Numeracy would be a better word to describe one's familiarity with numbers, one's ability to manipulate numbers or one's ability to crunch numbers. Mathematics, on the other hand, is about structures, describing structure, analysing structure and appreciating structure. Mathematics is sometimes perceived to be abstract as many of its concepts cannot be directly seen. However, what is making Mathematics so intriguing now is the fact that some of the abstract structures which have been developed over the years (developed as abstract structures for their own beauty and elegance) are now those very structures which describe the Quantum World. Abstract Mathematics is now the only tool available to explore, describe and manipulate the Quantum World, a real world. The question may be asked 'Is it proper to continue to call this mathematics abstract'? However, let us not get bogged down in semantics. It is worth pointing out that this mathematics, which is so accurate in describing the Quantum World, was initially perused for its own intrinsic beauty and elegance. Paul Dirac, who at the age of 31 years won the 1933 Nobel Prize in Physics, once wrote "It is more important to have beauty in one's equations than for the equations to fit experiment".[14]   Beauty and elegance have always been considered as a yardstick for the correctness of mathematics. Yet this beauty and elegance cannot be measured in any numerical way or to any degree of accuracy as the term accuracy is

---

[14]   http://en.wikipedia.org/wiki/Paul_Dirac

commonly known. A mathematician just knows that it is correct merely by its elegance. An elegant proof excites a mathematician. It makes them feel good.

2. The Mathematics Used in Describing the Quantum World

Plato, who was born in 427 BC and died in 347 BC, wrote:

> The reality which scientific thought is seeking must be expressible in mathematical terms, mathematics being the most precise and definite kind of thinking of which we are capable. [15]

It is clear Plato was not talking about numbers or merely the geometry of straight lines, curves and circles, nor about equations but more about mathematical thought which eventually led to such concepts as Groups, Rings, Fields, Vector Spaces etc.

We do not intend to go into any mathematical technicalities, but the reader might be interested in knowing the broad areas of mathematics which are used in describing and analysing the Quantum World. We can all remember the 'imaginary number', the square root of -1, which was introduced to us in secondary school. It is denoted by the letter 'i'. It is called imaginary because one cannot comprehend any number which when squared (multiplied by itself) gives the answer -1. Some would even go further and say that no such 'i' can exist as it is impossible to get a minus answer (<0) after squaring any number. And of course, that is correct if we limit ourselves to the Real Numbers. But if we expand the Real Numbers to include 'i', all multiples of 'i' and sums of these multiples with other Real Numbers, then we can build up

---

[15] http://plato.stanford.edu/entries/plato/

a whole new number system (the Complex Number system) and then explore the properties and characteristics of this new number system.

All of us were introduced to the circular functions of Sine, Cosine and Tangent in secondary school. In college days, some of us were introduced to that strange number called the Natural Number, denoted by the letter 'e' that has the approximate value of 2.718. The function $y=e^x$ (the Natural Exponential Function) has the peculiar property that when differentiated it remains unaltered. Some of us may also remember the hyperbolic functions which are defined in terms of the natural exponential and when first introduced do seem very strange, and a typical student often wonders what possible practical application these strange functions could have.

Well, it is these very same hyperbolic functions, together with the circular functions enveloped within the structure of a Vector Space over the Field of Complex Numbers that describe the Quantum World.[16] Any good student of mathematics will not be surprised to learn also that it is using the tools of Calculus within these structures that one is able to explore and analyse the Quantum World.

3.   The Fuzziness of the Quantum World[17]

But the most intriguing aspect of the Quantum World is the fuzziness and the uncertainty of anything in this world, and so it is here that the mathematical tools of Probability take centre stage.

---

[16]   Leonard Susskind, *Lecture Notes,* Stanford University, http://itunes.stanford.edu/
[17]   Leonard Susskind, *Quantum Theory Lectures,* Standford University, http://itunes.stanford.edu/

In the Quantum World, it is impossible to 'pin down' any 'object' or 'thing'. Rather than talk about an 'object' or a 'thing' in the Quantum World we talk about a photon. There is no common language which can adequately describe what a photon is. Objects, as we know them, have fixed properties like mass, however, a photon is mass-less. To oversimplify enormously, a photon is a tiny wave or particle of light. They are ideal for experiment as they can be seen as light and detected on an x-ray film. Photons and electrons behave in a very similar fashion. In talking about a photon, we will be using the term 'photon' to represent all other 'things' which exist in the Quantum World like an electron. It is impossible to have complete knowledge of a photon, that is to know its velocity and it position at any one time. Once its position is known, its velocity is unattainable and vice versa. Particular states (known position and known velocity of a photon) only potentially exist with specific probabilities. There is a specific probability attached to any potential existence. This 'fuzziness' makes many scientists uncomfortable and it does not fit the traditional moulds. However, as the English proverb says 'The proof of the pudding is in its eating', the proof of the real existence of the Quantum World is in the development of Quantum Computers. It is predicted that (for specific tasks and when fully developed) the computing power of one quantum computer will be greater than the combined computing power of all the computers presently in the world. The development of quantum computers is in its very early stages. However, there are crude versions of them in existence at present which tap into the potential contained in the Quantum World. We will say more about quantum computers in Chapter 7.

Chapter 6: Science and Quantum[18]

1.   Wave or Particle[19]

According to the understanding of the middle world, a wave and a particle are two different things and are governed by different laws. However, in the Quantum World a photon is both a particle and a wave at the same time or at least it behaves like a particle and a wave at the same time or some may say it behaves sometimes like a particle and sometimes like a wave. It is impossible to 'pin it down' to both position and velocity. So it is characterised by potential and possibility and probability. It is why we say there is a lot of fuzziness and uncertainty inherent in the Quantum World. Photons do not obey Newton's Laws of Motion or any other particular laws of the middle world.

2.   A Bundle of Energy in Relationship[20]

We cannot treat a photon as a mere particle. Probably, the strongest statement that can be made is that it cannot be isolated or, put it in another way, it exists only in relationship. Maybe relationship is how it can be defined or best described. We have to leave behind the standard notions of mass and motion and consider the possibility of describing a photon as 'a bundle of energy in relationship'. Are the building blocks of all of reality merely relationships of energy? The precise science of measurement and exactness seems to be totally inadequate to describe this reality of relationships of energy.

---

[18]   Marcus Chown, *Quantum Theory Cannot Hurt You*, Faber UK, 2007.
[19]   http://www2.slac.stanford.edu/vvc/theory/quantum.html
[20]   http://www.science.uwaterloo.ca/~cchieh/cact/c120/quantum.html

3.   Einstein's Theory of Relativity[21]

Taking the scientific and mathematical jargon out of the Theory of Relativity of Albert Einstein, basically the theory says that nothing exists in isolation but that everything depends on everything else. Notice how this differs greatly from the mechanical model where different parts are isolated and then analysed and examined. The Theory of Relativity (everything is relative) seems to correspond with much in the Quantum World. Einstein's famous equation $E=Mc^2$ where E denotes energy and M denotes mass while c is a constant (speed of light) is essentially saying that energy and mass are merely different faces of the same reality. This is far from our common notion of mass and energy. It seems, like the fish in the water that are unable to see (conceptualise) the whole lake, we too are limited in our vision. Our everyday language which is based on our everyday experience of reality is incapable of describing the bigger picture, the 'bigger lake' in which we live.

4.   Einstein and Mathematics

Mathematics can describe to some extent this 'bigger lake'. Einstein does so in mathematical terms using four-dimensional vector spaces and within this framework he is able to outline, predict and measure accurately the motion of stars and planets. The three-dimensional geometry which we all learned at school is not adequate to describe the time-space continuum which Einstein describes nor is it adequate to describe the 'curvature' of space which Einstein has shown is effected by the force of gravity. We, with our limited vision (like the fish in the water) see time and space as two different realities. Space, in our eyes, is fixed and time is continuously passing. However, it is not like that, it only

---

[21]   http://en.wikipedia.org/wiki/Theory_of_relativity.

appears to us (in our limited vision) to be like that. Time and Space are merely different faces of one reality. Science fiction films sometimes borrow from these concepts and to a strict rationalist these science fiction films may seem to be outrageously far from reality but in fact they may be far closer to reality than we may care to admit. We are now beginning to realise that during the past couple of centuries we have been exposed to an excess of rationalism which has blinded us to the bigger picture and to greater realities.

5.   The Mystics always had a Glimpse of these Realities

There has always been a strong connection between Philosophy, the Mystics and Mathematics. The Mystics, often with a strong philosophical background, merely by meditating, through silence and through stillness, have been able to come in touch with a deeper reality (deeper than the realities of the middle world which we experience with our five senses). Their writings on their experiences of these deeper realities are now corresponding with realities which are being discovered in quantum physics and quantum mechanics through the tools developed by mathematicians. And so now it is all beginning to come together, what the mystics say, what the scientists say and what the mathematicians say. Some of these convergences will be developed further in Chapter 8.

Chapter 7: Experiments in Science

1.   The Double Slit Experiment[22]

The Double Slit Experiment is a clear case where the rationality of Aristotelian logic breaks down completely. Here we see one photon going through two separate slits at the same time! One 'object' in two different places at the same time! This, in quantum terms, is referred to as 'a superposition of states'. And furthermore, after the one photon goes through two slits, its presence in two different places allows it (the single photon) to 'interfere' with itself and to act like a wave in motion! Our first reaction is disbelief. But remember the fish in the water; they cannot see the whole lake. Our minds are too small to see much of the bigger picture. Science is now inviting us to transcend the ordinary everyday picture of reality, to go beyond our everyday experience and to get a glimpse of the bigger picture.

2.   The Entanglement Experiment[23]

The concept of Entanglement opens up infinite possibilities of connectedness and relatedness. It has been proven that it is possible to connect or 'entangle' two photons in such a way that even if they are later separated by vast distances (even distances as large as light years), making a change to one photon will instantaneously effect the other photon. This 'entanglement' is completely beyond our understanding, yet it is real. It seems that reality will always be greater than what our minds can grasp. It is impossible for us to grasp how connected literally everything is. To bring out this connectedness and interconnectedness it is

---

[22]   http://www.doubleslitexperiment.com/
[23]   http://www.youtube.com/watch?v=BWyTxCsIXE4

symbolically (maybe realistically!) expressed in the idea that a butterfly flapping its wings in one of the rain forests in Misuku can have an effect on a tornado in Mexico![24] That is how related everything is. Again, the science based on isolating items is blown to pieces. Rather relationships and how things are related is the paramount issue if we are to have any proper understanding of reality. The scientist who cherishes interaction, inter-relatedness and connectedness is the one who will most probably reap the richest rewards and come to a fuller understanding of whatever he or she is seeking.

3.   No Such Thing as a Neutral Observer[25]

The most amazing aspect of the Double Slit Experiment is the effect on the experiment when the scientist tries to identify which slit the photon goes through. Observing the wave pattern of the single photon, it is clear that this single photon must pass through both slits. However, once the scientist actually looks at the photon passing through a slit, then it passes through only one slit!!! The photon ceases to act in a wave like manner and now acts as a pure particle, as a pure object of matter and once again obeys Newton's Laws of Motion! The act of observing changes the manner in which the photon behaves. So the idea that the observer can be neutral is also blown to pieces. There is no such thing as an objective or neutral observer. The observer scientist is actually himself/herself an integral part of the experiment. If the scientist wishes to see the photon act as a wave, it will act as a wave and if the scientist wishes to see the photon act as a particle, it will act like a particle. It depends on the observer scientist; whatever he or she wishes to see is what will be seen!

---

[24] James Gleich, *Chaos, Making a New Science*, Penguin New York, 1987.
[25] http://www.youtube.com/watch?v=DfPeprQ7oGc

4.   Quantum Computers[26]

The unbelievable phenomena of a single electron existing in two different places at one time and 'entangled' electrons acting in unison are now finding practical application in the middle world with the development of quantum computers. A classical computer has a memory made up of bits where each bit (an electrical charge) represents a '0' or a '1'. A quantum computer has memory made up of quantum bits, called qubits, where each qubit (an electron) can represent both a '0' **and** a '1' at the same time. Notice the emphasis on 'and'. This is possible because of the 'superposition of states'. The real computer power associated with quantum computing is seen when one considers that two qubits can represent all of four states simultaneously, three qubits can represent all of eight states simultaneously, four qubits can represent all of sixteen states simultaneously, ten qubits can represent all of one thousand and twenty-four states simultaneously while in the classical computer ten bits can only represent one state at any one time. Just imagine the number of states possible with 100 qubits! A whopping 2^{100} states! Since in the Quantum World one cannot observe directly an electron without interfering with it, scientists are circumventing this problem by looking at an 'entangled version' of the electron. This obviously is a simplification of all that is involved in the development of quantum computers which is very much in its infancy. But crude versions have been tested. In 2009 researchers at Yale University in New Haven, Connecticut, USA, created the first rudimentary solid-state quantum processor. The two-qubit superconducting chip was able to run elementary algorithms. Another team, working at the University of Bristol in the UK, also created a silicon-based quantum computing chip and was able to

---

[26]   http://www.sciencedaily.com/releases/2010/01/100110151331.htm

run Shor's Algorithm on the chip. Shor's Algorithm is an algorithm developed for quantum computing which factorises any number.[27]

5.   The Potential of Quantum Computers

Shor's Algorithm is important because it is expected that it will have the potential, using a quantum computer, to break the widely used public-key cryptography scheme known as RSA.[28] The security of the RSA cryptosystem is based on the assumption that factoring large numbers is computationally unfeasible. However, Shor's Algorithm shows that factoring is efficient on a quantum computer, so an appropriately large quantum computer can break the RSA cryptosystem. This large quantum computer is yet to be developed.

6.   Post Quantum Cryptography Research at Mzuzu University

Practically all present-day security in information, (in particular passwords or PIN numbers) is based on RSA type cryptography. So the development of quantum computers obviously has huge implications for e-commerce and banking institutions. It will render all RSA like cryptography useless. There is, however, another cryptosystem called the McEliece Cryptosystem, which is based on a family of Error Correcting codes called Goppa codes.[29] Many feel that this cryptosystem will withstand the power of quantum computing. The reader may be interested to know that Mzuzu University students and staff are in the forefront of researching this family of Goppa codes.

---

[27] http://en.wikipedia.org/wiki/Shor%27s_algorithm
[28] Douglas R. Stinson, *Cryptography; Theory and Practice,* CRC Press New York 1995.
[29] John A. Ryan, *Irreducible Goppa Codes,* PhD Thesis, University College Cork, Ireland, 2002.

Chapter 8: Implications of the New Science

1.   The Relatedness of Everything

Section 3 in Chapter 7 shows that the connections and relations between the observer scientist and the experiment are mind boggling. Again, we are thrown back on the relatedness and inter-relatedness of everything. In earlier chapters, we saw that nothing exists in isolation. All meaning is found in connectedness and inter-connectedness. It seems that the essential building blocks of everything can be described more in terms of waves of energy and an infinite sea of relationships rather than in terms of fixed matter. The well-known dictum 'no man is an island' now takes on new meaning. The electrons and protons and neutrons making up a chair and those making up my body are the same! The difference is in how they fit together and in how they are related to one another. Relationships are supreme. This too has implications for our own lives. It is the relationships which we cultivate which define us rather than 'the things' we possess.

2.   A Participatory World

The fact that the photon acts differently according to that which the observer scientist is seeking has very far reaching consequences. In classical science, the observer scientist is seen as neutral to the experiment having no effect on the outcome of the experiment. Indeed, this is one of the requirements for the experiment to be authentic in classical science. But in the Quantum World the observer scientist is involved in the experiment actually bringing about that which is being observed. The two positions could not be further apart. The whole question of a participatory world is now raised. We are not mere inhabitants of the world but we are participating in the on-going creation / development / transformation / evolution of the world to a far greater extent than we ever realised. This together with the fact that everything is connected and inter-connected makes us humans part of the whole movement towards transformation to higher realities. We are not spectators but deeply involved in the whole evolutionary process. Even without being consciously aware of it, we are involved but the exciting thing is that being aware allows us to be even more involved.

3.   Environmental Issues

Being aware brings us closer into the picture. Being aware gives us a greater respect for literally everything. We are now more conscious of how we depend on the environment and if we diminish the environment we diminish ourselves. Imagine what kind of mind we would have if we lived on the moon with no colour, no trees, and no animals, no anything! We too would be grey matter without any colour, without any imagination and without any creativity. It is imperative that we care for the earth, the trees, the fish, the animals, the hills, the valleys, the wetlands, the birds, the air, the rivers, the lakes, and not to forget the butterflies and all the rest. Matters of ecology are paramount in the preservation of live of all forms.

4.   The GAIA Hypothesis[30]

The GAIA hypothesis proposes that planet Earth has a life of its own. Like any life it needs sustenance. Like any life if it gets sick it can renew itself if given the space. But like any life, if it is not cared for and is overpowered by negative factors, it can die. We are coming to realise that we need planet Earth more than planet Earth needs us! Planet Earth can continue without us. In the past

---

[30]   James Lovelock, *A New Look at Life on Earth,* Oxford University Press, 1979.

planet Earth shook off the dinosaurs, maybe they were getting too big and too destructive of the environment. What about us humans now? Are we getting too destructive of the environment? Cancer, Swine Flu, HIV/AIDS, are these not the result of our 'miss-use' of the environment? Are we going to be shaken off planet Earth? We cannot survive without planet Earth. And so ecology comes into the equation. Care for the Earth comes into the equation. Environmental issues come into the equation. We are all in this together. We need each other.

5.   A New Mindset

A new mindset is required if we are to make sense of recent revelations in the Quantum World and related areas. We are enveloped by a universe of enormous diversity and vitality which is alive and pulsating. Everything is connected with everything else. We humans are not masters but rather co-creators. Practically nothing is predictable, rather we are being invited to be open to surprise, expectancy, wonder, creativity, beauty and elegance where the whole is greater than the sum of its parts. The human body which is extremely complicated, made up of so many forces and energies that we cannot comprehend fully, measure in any real way, observe with any great accuracy — like intimacy, the highs and lows of courtship, the excitement of sport, the exhilaration experienced on achievement, the terror of war or the anguish of the loss of a loved one. What is happening in the whole person cannot be analysed nor understood in terms of some of its parts. There is more to it than meets the eye. It is the same with all of reality; the real essence is deep within — more to do with relationships than with objects.

6.   New Revelation

Revelation now is not confined to the sacred books but creation as a whole is continually revealing the face of the divine. There has always been the notion that the beauty of nature reflected the beauty of the creator. However, traditionally, theology focused on the sacred books and on tradition. The world was seen as transitory and was not to be taken seriously. There was even the notion of fleeing *from the 'evil world'* in order not to be tainted by it. There is a shift now, especially with the insights of Evolution and Quantum Physics, we now know that the whole universe is just a massive expanding entity, a continuation of the Divine Creative Energy ever present. It is not transitory but part of the Kingdom of God and needs to be taken seriously. Our main function is to marvel and wonder at it all and to continue to sing and dance in unison with it.

7.   Redemption of All of Creation

In Christian circles, the three wise men coming to Bethlehem with gifts for the infant Jesus symbolise the universality of the implications of the Birth of Jesus for the whole human race, for peoples of all nations and all colours. Maybe, now with the greater understanding we have of the beginnings of the universe and the on-going creation of all that is, we may have a deeper understanding of what St Paul was pointing to when he said "not only we but the whole of creation is in one great act of giving birth".[31] Did St Paul have a glimpse of that possibility that Jesus came not only to save human beings but to save all of creation? Revelation seems to come to us bit by bit. In the Old Testament, there was a sharp awareness among the Israelites that God was on their side. The three wise men in the New Testament brought that

---

[31]   Romans 8:22

awareness to all peoples, that God is on the side of all peoples. Now, with the advance of knowledge, we are beginning to realise that the birth of Jesus has implications for all of creation. In this context, the first Chapter of the Gospel by St John is extremely rich:

> In the beginning was the Word:
> the Word was with God
> and the Word was God.
> He was with God in the beginning.
> Through Him all things came to be,
> no one thing has its being but through Him.

The implications are mind boggling. Who are we to limit the saving action of the Living God? The Dabhar was there before the beginning, there throughout the last 15 billion years and is there today continuing to redeem, to recreate and renew everything. Christmas is surely one mighty celebration of all of this. All that is left for us to do is to sing exultations of praise and glory which are best done in song and dance.

Chapter 9: Notes on Two Major Feasts of our Christian Heritage

Some of the major feasts of our Christian heritage gain deeper meaning from the recent discoveries in the scientific world. I cite two examples.

1. A Reflection on the Meaning of the Feast of the Epiphany

Epiphany, also Theophany or Three Kings' Day, is a Christian feast day that celebrates the revelation of God incarnate as Jesus Christ. In Christianity, the feast commemorates principally (but not solely) the visit of the Magi to the Christ child, and thus Jesus' physical manifestation to the Gentiles.[32] The Feast of the Epiphany is mainly seen as the extension of the promises (covenant) of God to the Israelites to all of humankind (Israelites and Gentiles). The 'Magi' were non-Israelites representing all who were not belonging to the Jewish Faith, the 'Gentiles'. With this event at the time of Jesus (visit of Magi to the child Jesus) the promise (covenant) of

---

[32] https://en.wikipedia.org/wiki/Epiphany_(holiday)

the Old Testament is extended to all peoples of all nations and so the promise becomes inclusive of all peoples.

What does 'EPIPHANY' mean for today's world? In the dictionary.com, Epiphany is defined as: 'a sudden, intuitive perception of or insight into the reality or essential meaning of something, usually initiated by some simple, homely, or commonplace occurrence or experience.'[33] I find this definition very enlightening ----Epiphany is the sudden intuitive perception after the visit of the Magi to the Child Jesus. With the increasing knowledge we have today of the unity of everything, this 'sudden intuitive perception' is extended. I suggest that the 'Feast of the Epiphany' has greater meaning than ever for the world of today. As observed in Section 3 of Chapter 8, we are part of the environment and the environment is part of us. We co-exist. Damage the environment and we damage ourselves. Promote the environment and we promote ourselves. It is not that we humans are 'separate from' the environment ---we are part of it. The environment is literally our breath, our air, our water, our inspiration, our colour, our life-line, etc. And remember the child Jesus was surrounded with animals, a donkey, a cow, sheep and he lay on straw/hay in a natural cave. And so the animals and the environment is all part of it. IT IS THE ENVIRONMENT WHICH NEEDS SALVATION. The environment includes 'us' and so if the environment is saved, we too are saved. The GAIA Hypothesis proposes that the whole planet Earth has a life of its own. The Epiphany extends the salvific act of the Child Jesus to this life of planet Earth. It is not just people! It is everything! It is planet Earth and even beyond! Pope Francis, in Laudato Si, says 'We are faced, not with two separate crises, one environmental and the other social, but with one complex crisis which is both social and

---

[33] http://www.dictionary.com/browse/epiphany.

environmental'[34] --- in other words, everything is together, unified, connected, integrated. It is only our illusionary perception that things are separated. I invite you to read Section 7 of Chapter 8, where I propose that redemption is for all creation. Epiphany is the celebration of that.

2. A Reflection on the Meaning of the Feast of the Trinity

Our forefathers in the Faith knew deep down that there was something special about the number 3 (trinity) and came to know God as three persons in relationship to one another. Science is now coming to the same conclusion about the number 3 and about relationships surrounding these three. The science of the quantum world is emphasizing that the 'building blocks' of the material world are not 'blocks' at all but rather 'relationships' or as stated in Section 2 of Chapter 6, 'bundles of energy in relationship'. A quark[35] is an elementary particle and a fundamental constituent of matter. Quarks combine to form protons and neutrons, the components of atomic nuclei. Quarks are never directly observed or found in isolation. Try to isolate a quark and it no longer exists! Quarks are only found in relationships with other quarks. And there are only three pairs of quarks! And so all material matter is made up of various relationships of a TRINITY of quark pairs! The focus is on relationships. The relationships are paramount and it is the relationships which give rise to matter. So the Feast of the Trinity is a celebration of relationships and a promotion of relationships which build a good world. We are challenged to develop relationships which build up. It is a time to ponder on the various relationships which we have, relationships between ourselves as people, relationships between ourselves and other non-human animal life, relationships between ourselves and plant

---

[34]   Laudato Si, Paragraph Number 139.
[35]   "Quark (subatomic particle)". *Encyclopaedia Britannica*, 2008.

life, relationships between ourselves and natural resources—in short relationships at all levels. It is a celebration and promotion of life in all its forms and in all its aspects. No wonder our forefathers put so much emphasis on the Feast of the Trinity.

Chapter 10: Our Response

1.   Celebrate through Rhythm and Dance

Movement, rhythm and dance are fundamental in the Quantum World. Literally everything is moving in an elegant dance. The electrons are in continuous motion around their nucleus. Atoms join up with other atoms, all in continuous rhythmic motion, to form molecules and molecules also have their own movement and dance. In the macro world, there is also movement and rhythm where the planets and stars are in continual motion, all performing their own dance. In the middle world, there seems to be an ingrained compulsion in all things towards dance. It is always a joy to witness animals dance as they express their spontaneity and creativity. We humans also delight in dance to music. Dance seems to touch something very deep in us as if it is fundamentally a part of us. Maybe it is why pop stars like Michael Jackson make such an appeal to us all. We seem to get mesmerised by the spontaneity and rhythm of their elegant movements. We seem to get carried away to a new plane, to new horizons as we become part of the dance. Initially one tries to synchronise one's body movements with the music of the dance and then it is as if the dance takes over and we are then moved spontaneously by the dance itself.[36] We are carried by the dance and its energy, whether bodily or in mind, to a state of unity and wholeness, yet within a freedom of spontaneity and seemingly ordered chaos, to a place of ecstasy. This is why dance is so appropriate for celebrating that Divine Creative Intelligence, Creative Wisdom, Creative Energy, which was there in the beginning, there throughout all of the billions of years of history of the universe, continually creating, continually shaping, continually transforming and still there now,

---

[36] Diarmud O'Murchu, *Quantum Theology* , Crossroad Publishing, New York, 2004, Chapter 4.

continuing to create, shape and transform everything. And this dance, once we synchronise ourselves to it, makes us part of the same movement towards the creation of a new world and the transformation of all that is. Gladly, this dance is still an integral part of African liturgy, African worship and African celebration. This is one of the many areas where Africa can enrich the rest of the world.

2.   Mathematics Having the Final Word

It is appropriate in this paper for Mathematics to have the final word. It is interesting to mathematicians that this rhythm, this music, this dance can also be captured somewhat in mathematical structures. Within the music and the dance there is symmetry. Symmetry is always connected to harmony and simplicity and beauty. It was in the pursuit of this beauty in symmetry that the mathematical structure of Group Theory developed. Now with the advent of Algorithmic Mathematics and with the power of computing, this symmetry can be generated into computer images. This is what is becoming to be known as Fractal Geometry. It is far from the dots, straight lines and curves of Euclidean Geometry but exploits the ordered chaos and the unseen symmetry in nature and captures it in a mathematical algorithm form, which can be run on computer. The variety of possibilities in algorithmic form is vast, which reflects the true nature of things in the natural world. Again, we see the wisdom of Plato when he declared that

> The reality which scientific thought is seeking must be expressible in mathematical terms, mathematics being the most precise and definite kind of thinking of which we are capable.[37]

---

[37] http://en.wikipedia.org/wiki/Plato.

The Question of God and Evolution

Introduction

Stephen Hawking[1] and Roger Penrose[2] are among the present world experts on the beginnings of the cosmos, black holes and evolution in general. They have worked together on the well-known publication *"The Nature of Space and Time"*[3]. However, they differ on the question of whether there is a place for God in the evolution of all of that exists. Stephen Hawking argues that the universe is self-contained and has its own dynamic in the continuing process of evolution[4]. Roger Penrose argues that it is not helpful to exclude the possibility of a God from the process of evolution.[5] In this piece we try to delve into the question of not

---

[1]   www.hawking.org.uk.
[2]   http://cajal.unizar.es/eng/part/Penrose.html
[3]   http://www.friesian.com/penrose.htm
[4]   http://www.universetoday.com/79294/steven-hawking/
[5]   http://cajal.unizar.es/eng/part/Penrose.html

only the possibility of the existence of God in the beginning of evolution and in the ever-on-going process of evolution but also what it means to say that God exists in it all. Let us begin by reviewing what many traditions and religions mean when they talk about God.

An attempt to put human language on the concept of God

Theology has always claimed that God cannot be captured in human terms and certainly not in human language. However, even though God is beyond all our imaginings, our grasp, our language, we have no other medium to try to grasp the reality that is God. We have no alternative but to try to put words on it. Maybe the best we can do is to try to expound on the different aspects of God and try to shed some light on that which is infinite. So, we make an attempt.

In many traditions, the following attributes are often given to God:[6]

- God is eternal. God has always existed, has no beginning, no origin, no source, has always been there and will always be there.

- God is the creator of everything. God is seen as the source of everything, the creator of all that is. Everything that exists owes its existence to God.

- God is sovereign, that is God rules over all of history.

---

[6] http://atheism.about.com/od/doesgodexist/u/ Atheolo-gyReligionCriticism.htm#s2

- God is provident, that is God acts in history, guides the course of history and is in control of everything.

- God is personable. It is possible to have a real personal relationship with God. It is possible for people to communicate with God. It is possible for God to communicate with people.

- God cares for all of creation. God wishes that all of creation flourishes.

- God is perfection itself. God lacks nothing.

- God is everywhere. The presence of God is all pervasive, not only in people but in all things and in all places.

- God is omnipotent, that is all powerful. This follows from the belief that God has always been there, is the creator of everything and is perfect.

- God is omniscient, that is all knowing. There is nothing beyond the knowledge of God.

- God is omnibenevolent, that is God is all caring and all nurturing. God wishes the best for every person and every created thing.

- God is transcendent and immanent. These two seem to our little human minds to be in contradiction but the idea that God is greater than everything and the idea that God is intimately involved in everything do coexist together.

- God is infinite. God is beyond our understanding.

- God is immutable. God cannot change. God is always the same.

It may also help to list a few ideas about God which are unhelpful, ideas which lead us in the wrong direction, ideas which eventually bring us into conflict with other branches of knowledge and so we also attempt to say what God is not. Among other things:

- God is not external to this planet.

- God is not primarily sitting in judgment on peoples' lives.

- God does not suspend natural processes in a miraculous or supernatural way

Belief in the Presence of God

Those who believe in the existence of God often declare that God is everywhere, present in all things, especially present in people and, in particular, present in those who are open to Him and who believe in Him. Believers are convinced that this presence is all pervasive, that it is active and effective and that it makes a difference in peoples' lives. Believers are also convinced that this presence is everlasting, has been there always, is there now and will be there in the future.

Trying to Rationalize the Presence of God

However, when one tries to 'pin down' this presence or 'locate it in a definite way', one runs into difficulties. Any attempt to 'pin down' this presence is an attempt to bring it under the rationalizing processes which have gone on over the last couple of centuries in scientific circles.

Interestingly, quantum physicists also encounter the same problem when they try to 'pin down' the existence of quarks, electrons and photons.[7] Just as there is no adequate language to describe 'God', there is no common language which can adequately describe what a photon is. Objects, as we know them, have fixed properties like mass, however a photon is mass-less! To oversimplify enormously, a photon is a tiny wave or particle of light. They are ideal for experiment as they can be seen as light and detected on an x-ray film. Photons and electrons behave in a very similar fashion. We can use the term 'photon' to represent all other 'things' which exist in the Quantum World like electrons and quarks. It is impossible to have complete knowledge of a photon or an electron, that is, to know its velocity and its position at any one time. Once its position is known, its velocity is unattainable and vice versa. Particular states (known position and known velocity of a photon) only potentially exist with specific probabilities. There is a specific probability attached to any potential existence. This 'fuzziness' makes many scientists uncomfortable and it does not fit the traditional moulds.

A New Language

This language of the 'fuzziness' of the quantum world does suit better to shed light on the existence of God. This existence cannot be pinned down, it is everywhere and it cannot be predicted. So the quantum world is now giving us a language to better express the 'everywhereness' of God and a language to understand better that God cannot be contained in anything and yet is contained in everything. Once you try to isolate a quark in the quantum world, it no longer exists. A quark only exists in relation to other quarks. Yet everything is made up of quarks!

---

[7]   Marcus Chown, *Quantum Theory Cannot Hurt You*, Faber UK, 2007.

Now we are beginning to realize that we have tried to rationalize too many things and that not everything can be subjected to the rational arguments of what we term 'objective science'. In fact objective science itself is now coming to the realization that not everything obeys Newton's Laws of Motion, not everything follows the laws of logic as espoused by the empirical sciences and that in general there has been far too much rationalizing of everything. The well-known 'Double Slit Experiment' in Quantum Physics is an eye opener.

The Double Slit Experiment and Openness to Mystery

The well-known "Double Slit Experiment"[8] in Quantum Physics demonstrates in a laboratory the fact that a single photon can go through two different slits or holes simultaneously, thus demonstrating that the quantum (microscopic) world behaves in a very different way from the world which we live in and which we experience every day. Philosophers have for many centuries been in touch with the fact that the material world we live in, is merely an illusion, a concept of our own making, and have been asking difficult questions about what really does exist or even if anything at all exists and they have been asking these questions for a long time now. The mystics too, down through the ages, have come to know that a deeper reality lies behind all that is known as the material world, they have got in touch with this deeper reality through silence and contemplation and they usually emerge completely transformed. In every age there have been people who were able to discern a spiritual dimension within the material world, have been able to somehow connect to this spiritual dimension and communicate something of this spiritual dimension to others. Many of these people would be known under such

---

8   http://www.doubleslitexperiment.com/

names as gurus, holy men or holy women or faith healers. It seems
to me that those scientists, who are open to mystery, are now
coming to the same conclusions as the philosophers, the mystics,
the gurus, the holy women, the holy men and the faith healers.
Some scientists would vehemently object, saying that they do not
see any connection between spirituality and science. It is possible
that some scientists (not all), in coming to such conclusions, are
operating out of a reduced view of spirituality, an impoverished
version of religion and a magical interpretation of the divine. For
an authentic vision of God, one would now need to integrate the
concept of a living God with the on-going process of evolution,
rather than see God as an extra, added-on reality, external to
everything that exists. If it is a God who is outside the created
universe and if heaven is some place/state external to the cosmos,
then many of the long list of attributes generally given to God
above would not apply.

Further New Language of the Double Slit Experiment

The "Double Slit Experiment" mentioned above literally opens up
infinite vistas, open-ended possibilities and never-ending potential.
Imagine one thing existing simultaneously in two places, three
places, four places...!!! This is not mere science fiction but it is
proven and observed by scientific experiment in a laboratory. This
can be described by the term bi-location or better still non-location
emphasizing the fact that the photon has no fixed position or
location. But it is best described as potentially existing in many
different places. Here the mathematical tools of probability take
center stage together with the concept of a vector space over the
field of the complex numbers. I have listened to hours of lectures
of Leonard Suskind on YouTube detailing the mathematics which
describe this potential existence in various places. The beauty and
the elegance of the mathematics involved verifies the truth of the

reality. This non-locality and potential existence in the Quantum World, does it not mirror our belief, our knowledge, our conviction that God is not confined to any location or particular place, our knowing that God can potentially exist anywhere? We have always used our everyday experience (it is the only thing we can use) of the world to try to shine light on and to express the deeper realities of Faith and of God. Now that our everyday experience of the world is changing, now that we are beginning to see the world in a new way, now that we are gaining more insight into the realities that exist, we may use these new insights, a new understanding of things which exist in order to shed more light on and in order to give greater expression to the deeper realities which lie behind that facade of things which we see with our eyes. The non-locality or the potential existence of things at the quantum level does give a language for the greater expression of the idea that God is everywhere, or at least that He is potentially everywhere.

Energy and Matter

One of the great discoveries of Einstein is that matter and energy are essentially different faces of the same thing demonstrated by the equation $E=Mc^2$ where 'c' is a constant, 'E' stands for energy while 'M' stands for mass.[9] For the non-mathematician let me emphasise the implication of this equation. Since "c" is a constant (does not change) essentially $E=M$, i.e. energy is mass (matter). For our small minds matter is something fixed, solid-like, unchangeable, static, it is just there, while energy is something alive, moving, active, being expended and continually being changed. It is just our perception of it, but really 'matter' and 'energy' are the same! So everything is energy! Everything is in

---

[9] http://en.wikipedia.org/wiki/Theory_of_relativity

motion. Everything is connected. It is only that we perceive things to be separate. But nothing is really separate. Now this throws us back to the philosophers and the mystics who from time way back knew these things. It is fascinating that science is now coming to the same conclusion. As the English proverb says 'there are many ways to kill a cat' there are also many different ways of approaching the mystery which underlies all of reality. I am afraid to say that Science is not the latest arrival, as there have been many scientists and many mathematicians throughout history who did have a unified and integrated approach to scientific rigor and spirituality. But in general, in the public view, Science and Belief in God did seem to clash. Now it is becoming more apparent that there is no clash.

Lines of Energy and Lines of Connectedness

In a recent booklet named *Science and Spirituality*[10] we have talked about spheres of connectedness. There is a very interesting phenomenon which is only recently coming to light. There are lines of energy and lines of connectedness and lines of communication in operation of which we know very little of. For example, some years back, crows in America started dropping nuts on the highways in front of cars in order to crack the hard outer shells and easily eat the soft centres. Around the same time crows in Japan started the same behaviour. Was this merely a coincidence? Are there lines of energy or communication operational between crows of which we are not in tune with? It would be very difficult for us to deny such a possibility. There is another story told of twins who were living on different continents. One of the twins, while he was working in a factory, accidently got his arm cut off and at that moment the other twin, on a different continent,

---

[10]   Mzuni Press, 2011.

roared in pain. What lines of energy were operational? Energy is all around us. People talk about fields of energy and spheres of energy. How are these spheres and fields impinging on us? It is clear that the Field of Gravity is keeping our feet firmly on the ground. It is clear that the Electromagnetic Field, present all over the earth, allows us to speak on our cell phones to anywhere on earth where there is a network established. Doctors and healers are aware of energy levels surrounding a person and sometimes are able to manipulate these spheres of energy for healing purposes. The power of positive thinking on the wellbeing of a person is well recognized. Many have no problems in asserting the flow of energy within a person but hesitate when we talk about the flow of energy between different persons. Is this because of our illusion of separateness? Is it because of our reluctance to see the connectedness of everything?

The universe began with a big bang, a big burst of energy and this energy is continuing to burst out, to expand, to evolve and to create anew. All energy came from that Big Bang and so in that sense all energy is connected. And let's remember that everything is energy! This dynamic view of reality is far from the static view of former times when it was once thought that way back at some instance in the distant past the universe was created once and for all time. We are now more aware that everything is in continual motion, continually changing, continually evolving, continuing to be created.

Back to the Holy Men, Holy Women and Mystics

One of the common attributes given to God in the Christian context is that God is a person. This does not mean that God has a nose, a mouth, teeth, legs, hands etc. Neither does it say He hasn't! But what it definitely does say is that it is possible to relate to God, to listen to Him, to speak to Him, to communicate with Him and to have a personal relationship with Him. The mystics, the holy men and the holy women are able to do this. By communicating with God, they are changed themselves and are able to effect change in others. Belief and Faith in a personal God is powerful. It has the power to transform. And that is exactly what God is doing with everything, transforming not just people but literally transforming everything. Why limit God's action, God's transforming power to people? As St Paul says "He is bringing everything together under Christ as Head, everything in the heavens and everything on earth." This brings us to the question of the meaning of Christ in the context of evolution. Pierre Teilhard de Chardin wrote excitingly about the 'Cosmic Christ' as he saw all of evolution bringing everything together under the 'Cosmic Christ' as the 'Omega Point' and at the same time all things emanating from Christ and everything being created in and through Him, as the 'Alpha Point'. Christ is the Alpha and the Omega of all of evolution. However, this whole concept of Christ as the Cosmic Christ is too large for these few pages and is worth many papers of its own.

A Poor Attempt at Describing the Reality that is God

Any attempt to describe God is very inadequate. However, we have no choice but to try. With the foregoing discussion on quantum things and the new science of the quantum world and the new knowledge contained in the new science of evolution and the new language which all of this brings, we are able to make a better attempt at expressing the infinity which is contained in God. If we understand that transforming spirit, that creative spirit, that transcending spirit which is contained in everything, pushing everything to greater heights, transforming everything to new levels, that all pervasive impulse which is projecting everything to greater complexity as the Spirit of the Living God, as that Divine Presence among us, as that Divine Creative Energy there from the beginning and still here today, in short as the living God among us, then we may read all those attributes given to God in a new light. In the light of the above these attributes take on new freshness. We again list the attributes and comment on each in the light of the foregoing discussion.

- "God is eternal. God has always existed, has no beginning, no origin, no source, has always been there and will always be there." Yes, there was the Big Bang nearly 15 billion years ago but where did that singularity at time zero of the Big Bang come from? Scientists agree they can never know anything about time zero as the laws of physics do not apply there! It is simply impossible to 'pin down' the 'time zero' moment.

- "God is the creator of everything. God is seen as the source of everything, the creator of all that is. Everything that exists owes its existence to God." Now, with evolution, we are coming to understand how dynamic creation is and how it is all continuing at all times. With our new understanding of the Divine Presence in it all, it gives fresh meaning to the on-going process of creation. We are awe stricken with the thought that we actually are partners with God in this on-going creation!

- "God is sovereign, that is God rules over all of history. Since He is the one who is the driving force behind it all, the transforming force bringing everything to new levels, to greater complexity, to greater consciousness, He is the One who is ruling and guiding everything.

- "God is provident, that is God acts in history, guides the course of history and is in control of everything." The concept of Evolution and the idea of the presence of the Divine Active Creative Spirit transforming everything makes it easier to see how God is Provident and how He is actively shaping everything and how He acts in time and history.

- "God is a personable. It is possible to have a real personal relationship with God. It is possible for people to communicate with God. It is possible for God to communicate with people." The recent advances in quantum physics reveal the existence of hitherto unknown connections and relatedness. The spheres of energy which abound all around us open up infinite possibilities for communicating with and relating to that which sustains everything. The possibility of getting in touch with that spirit which underlies everything and guides everything is made more real. The fact that everything cannot be explained by scientific logic is refreshing. There is more room for God to exist! There are more possibilities for communication with a deeper reality. Lines of communication exist of which we know very little. The fact that the mystics got in touch with a deeper reality underlying all that is visible is a strong indication that such lines of communication do exist.

- "God cares for all of creation. God wishes that all of creation flourishes." This is exactly what is happening in evolution! All things are being transformed to new levels, to more complexity and to greater consciousness. It is the Spirit of God which is driving all to their final goal in realizing their transcendence. Everything is being brought together under

Christ as head, everything in the heavens and everything on earth.

- "God is perfection itself. God lacks nothing." Since evolution is about continual change and the idea of perfection has connotations of being static, it is more difficult to place this attribute within the context of the evolution of all that there is. In the context of evolution, it is even difficult to grasp what the idea of perfection means. Perfection itself is part of evolution and is also being transformed all the time. But if we take perfection to mean continual transformation to more complex and more conscious states then the idea of perfection fits the concept of evolution in a better way and such an attribute of perfection can easily be applied to God as the author and sustainer of evolution.

- "God is everywhere. The presence of God is all pervasive, not only in people but in all things and in all places." This attribute becomes alive in evolution since God is the spirit driving everything to transformation, to greater consciousness, to new levels. In this context God is obviously in all things and everywhere.

- "God is omnipotent, that is all powerful." The concept of evolution together with the belief that God is the Creative Spirit behind everything places the power of God at the heart of everything. When talking about the power of God we are not talking about the power for God to perform arbitrary acts but rather God works within the framework of evolution and being omnipotent means that within that framework nothing is beyond Him. He is the one who is doing the transforming and the evolving and the bringing of everything to greater consciousness.

- "God is omniscient, that is all knowing. There is nothing beyond the knowledge of God." Some way or another, that Creative and Transforming Spirit, which is ever operative in history, seems to know where everything is heading. This brings a great peace of mind to the believer who can celebrate this omniscience and give praise and thanks for it.

- "God is omnibenevolent, that is God is all caring and all nurturing. God wishes the best for every person and every created thing." In evolution, the benevolence of God is more clearly seen as all things are being taken to a higher level, to greater complexity, to greater consciousness, to a greater unity, to a greater coherence, to a greater integration—in short to a new life.

- "God is transcendent and immanent. These two seem to our little human minds to be in contradiction but the idea that God is greater than everything and the idea that God is intimately involved in everything have coexisted together." The idea of the hologram in science and of fractals in mathematics is now bringing to the fore the idea that not only is the whole (the complete thing) more than the sum of its parts but even the whole is contained in each of its parts.[11] Again the language of the scientists is coming close to the language of the philosophers, theologians and mystics. To those who are open to it, the new language of evolution and quantum physics is allowing us to give greater expression to the deeper spiritual realities within us and within all of reality. The formulation of such an expression is bringing God to a greater consciousness within all of reality which is itself part of the evolutionary process.

---

[11] *Science and Spirituality*, Mzuni Press, 2011.

This very formulation is itself a powerful tool in driving all things to greater consciousness.

- "God is infinite. God is beyond our understanding." Mathematics has, since the time of George Cantor, delved into the mysteries of infinity and infinities. Mathematics distinguishes between an infinity, an infinity of infinities, an infinity of infinities of infinities, and so on.... And there is no end to it. And when the vastness of it all is brought before our minds, a greater expression is given to the concept of infinity, and to the concept of God. In making this greater expression we are making the reality more real and more conscious. In this way, we are actively participating in the whole process of evolution.

Conclusion

Science and Spirituality are coming closer together. The science of evolution and the science of the quantum world is giving new language which facilitates the attempt to express the in-expressible. Science and Spirituality both gain from interacting with one another, they enrich one another as ultimately they speak of the same reality. A greater realization of the connectedness and inter-connectedness of everything is now beginning to dawn on the scientist, the mystic, the holy woman, the holy man, the philosopher or whatever you may call the spiritual person. This connectedness and inter-connectedness is opening up exciting possibilities for Science and Spirituality and Religion to interact for the benefit of all.

Printed in the United States
By Bookmasters